# My Sisters Guide to Keto:
## Advice from Someone Who's Been There

# My Sister's Guide to Keto:
## Advice from Someone Who's Been There

**SHEREETA VANVLEET**

My Sister's Keto
2019

First Printing: 2019

ISBN 978-0-359-53878-2

My Sister's Keto
4708 Steinbeck APT 201
Ames, IA 50014

U.S. trade bookstores and wholesalers: Please contact My Sister's Keto

 Tel: (317) 360-8877; or email mysistersketo@outlook.com.

www.mysistersketo..com

# Dedication

Dedicated to Courtney and Mariah: You guys are the best part of my life. You both have taught me that while being a sister is nice, being a mom is so much better! I love you, my beautiful girls

# Contents

Preface .............................................................................. ix

Introduction ...................................................................... 2

Chapter 1: Get Your Mind Right................................... 9

Chapter 2: So…What is Keto Anyway??? ...................... 15

Chapter 3: How Do We Get Started on Keto?...................... 23

Chapter 4: What Do We Eat on Keto? ...................... 35

Chapter 5: Ready, Set, Go!!! ...................................... 45

Chapter 6: Weight Loss ................................................ 51

Chapter 7: Intermittent Fasting.................................... 58

Chapter 8: Supplements................................................ 62

Chapter 9: Keto FAQ's ................................................ 64

# Preface

*To proclaim the favorable year of the Lord and the day of venge-ance of our God; To comfort all who mourn, to grant those who mourn in Zion, giving them beauty for ashes*
    *Isaiah 62:1-3*

Yes, He said He would give us beauty for ashes…but in order to get ashes, some things have to burn. It's time to let go of our old mind-sets, beliefs, habit and let them burn so that we may see the beauty beneath

I am not a medical doctor or provider, and I have the utmost respect for the work that medical professionals provide. This book is in no way to be used to diagnose any condition nor should it be used to cure any disease processes.

# Introduction

I never thought that I would actually write a book. Not because I wasn't capable, but I'm just being honest. Although I've lived an interesting life so far, nothing seemed to merit the writing of a book...not until I was faced with the fact of my very life being in peril due to the poor health and food choices that I was making. So, while there are probably other stories I could tell, nothing really could be compared to the story of how I had to pull myself together and recommit to my health through Keto. Today, I have succeeded in assisting others in committing themselves to better health through the adjustment of their eating habits, and it has completely become my passion project. Through the lessons I've learned, I am now committed to sharing my story, and I'm hoping to empower and inspire someone else out there who may feel as though all hope is lost because of the physical and emotional pain of being overweight and the health issues associated with it. Many people believe that pain is just a part of their existence and that's all there is to it. It absolutely does not have to be that way. I'm going to spare you most of the gory details of my existence and just focus on one main thing, my journey on Keto and giving you the best advice on how to successfully start this lifestyle.

I stumbled on Keto during the summer of 2018. I was in so much physical and emotional pain that I would have tried just about any diet...and I did! For the two years prior to the summer of 2018, I was able to "fake the funk" and keep everything on the exterior of my life looking fine. However, I was emotionally lost on the inside. My decline began with the lifestyle changes of leaving the U.S Army after 20 years of service, going back to college to finish my degree, and then taking a job at a well-known computer company; it all sounds great on the surface, but I managed to gain 100lbs during that short time span, which is not healthy. Although, I tried working out feverishly, no matter how many miles I ran, or weights I lifted, I could not outwork my horrible diet. The harder I worked, the more discouraged and depressed I became because the weight would not come off. I started to doubt myself and developed a horrible case of imposter syndrome. Whether at work or at home, I felt like a complete failure. At work, I was under a lot of pressure, most of which was self-induced. It was my first "real" job outside of the military and college, and I wanted to prove that I could be successful. I was working hard and performing as expected, but I always felt like someone was going to discover that I didn't belong there, and I would lose everything. The more anxious I became, the more I ate. I was allowed to telecommute from home, and when my husband was away at work, I was free to cook (and eat) huge breakfasts that could have fed two people. My favorite was smothered potato hash browns with corned beef hash and butter toast, along with 2 cans of cream soda. I'd wait for my husband to leave for work, I'd make my meal, and eat while I was on conference calls. No matter how much I ate, I could not get full.

It seemed that nobody really noticed. No matter how much I was eating and gaining, nobody seemed to notice or care. Nobody ever commented on my weight or suggested that maybe I seek help. As long as I was performing as expected, it was all good…but it wasn't. Again, on the outside, I had the handsome, attentive husband, but inside our home, things were chilly. I began to snore so loudly that it was hard for him to even sleep in the same room with me. I was so uncomfortable in my skin that I never wanted to be naked, especially in front of him, even him touching me was out of the question. I hated myself. When we met, I was in such great shape, I was so outgoing and full of life but, as my depression deepened, I withdrew away from him, and my frustration and anger at myself spilled over into our relationship and into the relationship I had with my daughters.

In a matter of 24 months, my life seemed to unravel, and things started to take a turn for the worse. My health declined swiftly. I began to suffer from acid reflux and constant heart burn. My lower back, legs and feet would hurt all the time. Even standing at the sink to wash the dishes was so painful that I would be frustrated and yell at my daughters for leaving dishes in the sink. I became an unpleasant person to be around, and I could not seem to get my life together. The part that bothered me the most about all of it was that it wasn't always this way for me.

The wall in my home office is full of plaques, certificates, awards, my degree, and other trinkets and mementos from my time in the military and volunteering around the various communities that I had lived. I call it "the wall of accomplishment". I'd look at it and read over the details listed on the certificates, from time to time, trying to restoke the fire in my brain. It seemed like I was always in a fog and I seem not to be able to get back to the woman described on the plaques hanging on the wall.

One of the best parts of Keto, in my opinion, is being able to be that woman again, in fact, I feel like a more powerful version of her. If I had to choose between the weight loss and regaining my cognitive function, I would choose the mental clarity, cognitive function, and stabilized moods, hands down.

# My Sister's Keto

I started My Sister's Keto after I began to win the fight to get my life back. As I began to learn about Keto and go through the process of cutting out the sugar, processed foods and reducing my carbohydrate intake down to the recommended amount, the differences began to show up almost immediately in my life. During my first week of Keto I'd lost 8 pounds, and in a month, I'd lost 14 pounds. My mental clarity had improved so much. It was as if I'd been driving through the worst fog and the sun appeared to burn it all away to reveal the clearest sunny day my eyes had ever seen! I was sold! Whenever anyone asks me, to this day, I tell them I am never going back to eating sugar and processed foods. It is now my mission to aid anyone looking to learn how to start positively improving their lives through mindful nutrition (Keto), hydration, and exercise.

Many people have asked me, "Why did you name your company 'My Sister's Keto'?" and the answer to that question is simple. I am a sister and have been in the entire sense of the word for the entirety of my life. I am my mother's oldest child, my sister and I are barely 15 months apart in age, and up until I was 18 years old, we never spent any real time apart. The day after I turned 18, I went to the U.S. Army recruiting office in Indianapolis, Indiana and made the decision that would be the cornerstone of my entire adult life. I proudly served as an enlisted member of the Army for 20 years. During that time, often, my role was that of a big sister. As a noncommissioned officer, my job was to train and lead soldiers, many of them young and in need of guidance.

I took my role very seriously, and I worked tirelessly to learn the tenants of leadership, motivating people, and the characteristics of the type of leader that people would feel comfortable approaching and taking instruction from. If a soldier needed a word of advice, a compassionate ear, or a swift kick in the butt, I was there to provide for them. I kept myself in great physical condition so that I could hang with my younger troops during physical training. In fact, it seemed like the older I got, the better I got. During much of my career, I worked extremely hard to be able to execute forced foot marches with a 35-pound ruck sack on my back. I could run for miles without complaint; in fact, I'd run several Army 10-mile races and had a great time doing it! Except for when I gave birth to my daughters, I pretty much kept myself in great physical condition. I wanted to set the example for any soldier that was around me. I wanted to do it all and show my soldiers that it could be done. I truly felt that this was my purpose in life; to provide good training, guidance, mentorship, and to be a leader. I was good at it, and I was able to build relationships that stand to this day.

Once I retired from the Army in December of 2015, I must admit, I took for granted that my physical condition would not really change much. As Mike Tyson once said, you always have a plan until you get punched in the face, and life seemed to be punching me dead in the face. It is my mission now, to help those who are getting punched in the face. I don't ever want any of you to feel that you are alone, or don't have anyone who will notice you and understand your pain. No matter how successful you are in one part of your life, there can still be pain, dysfunction and poor health in other parts. The goal of this book is to speak life into your situation, to motivate you, and to teach you how to incorporate the Keto way of eating into your life so that you can find the health, physical wellbeing, and mental clarity you deserve.

# Chapter 1: Get Your Mind Right

*For as a man thinketh in his heart so is he – Proverbs 23:7*

It's been said about me, my entire life, "Once Shereeta makes her mind up about something…"

There are times where my resolve may come off as a bit stubborn or like I'm trying to be hard headed but it's something that has served me well in my life. When I make a decision about something, it is not taken lightly. I make proper research on my decision, weigh my options and give it lots of thought. Sometimes, like in the case of my weight loss journey, it can take me a while to finally make my mind up BUT, once the decision gets made, that's it!

Before the day that I finally made my mind up that I was truly ready to change my lifestyle and make my health a priority, there were a lot of false starts. I would get excited about embarking on a new diet or fitness class. I would buy new workout clothes and shoes. I would buy fat burners, energy pills, and "get lean quick" pills. I drank all kinds of teas and green drinks. I tried waist trainers with "special" lotions to help me sweat. I tried limiting my calories to insanely low limits, eating low fat, and I tried all the special diet superfoods and shakes. I could go a good week, but at the end of that week, I'd be starving for my cheat meal - a reward for being so "good". That cheat meal was usually saved for a Friday, and that one meal would turn into an entire weekend of treats. That weekend would spill over into the next week and that ultimately turned into another failed attempt, which turned into another thing to beat myself up about, "why am I such a failure?".

I wish that I could go back in time and tell that woman that she is NOT a failure. I would beg her to not be so hard on herself; she deserves much better than that! This world can be a cold hard place by itself, and she doesn't need to add to that. This brings me to my first piece of sisterly advice:

**The first piece of sisterly advice is GET YOUR MIND RIGHT!**

None of us would allow anyone to talk to us (or about us) the way that we have talked to (or about) ourselves! Self-doubt is the killer of dreams, goals, and aspirations. Instead of letting self-doubt and negative self-talk kill our dreams, we need to kill it first. The truth is this: It doesn't matter how many times you read this book, you could even buy 1000 copies of it. You could buy the best running shoes on the market. You can have the best of everything but, until you decide in your mind and in your heart that you will be successful, healthy and whole – you will fail. You must resolve in yourself that you will not let yourself kill your health and fitness goals. I would say I'm lucky because once I (finally) made my mind up, that was it. At the time, I was so desperate to change my circumstances; it wasn't hard to get firm in my decision. I wanted my life, my marriage, my body and my health back! I was willing to fight for it.

You must, once and for all, commit yourself to your health. You have to believe that you can do what needs to be done, understanding that it doesn't have to be done all in one swoop or one day. The process of healing yourself from the inside out takes time. Like many of you, I too would be on fire to start something, but if I didn't see immediate results it had to either be that it wasn't for me or that I wasn't doing it right. Even as I'm writing this line right now, I chuckle to myself about how silly that notion is. Look, It's about process and progress, NOT PERFECTION. As you begin your Keto journey, you must believe that you can be successful, then trust the process, and make note of your progress as you go. Remember, none of us got to where we are (fat and in poor health) in a day, so it's going to take us longer than a day to find our way back to good health.

As you begin to become firm in your resolve to lose weight and regain your health through Keto, you're going to have to work on your focus. There will have to be a part of you that says, "Even though I don't see it yet, I know it's coming!", and lean on that. I promise you, that very phrase has been a part of my mantra since day one. I made a conscious effort to walk with my head up, shoulders back and faith on high as if I'd already lost every last ounce I wanted to lose.

As I made the changes to my diet, I also started making changes in my mind. I began to act as if I had already reached my goal. I smiled more, I looked people in the eye, and I started leaving my house more, Prior to that point, I had been isolating myself, too ashamed to let people in because of how far I thought I'd fallen. Once I'd made up my mind, I also changed my focus. Instead of focusing on how much weight I'd gained, I focused on my great comeback story. It was not easy, but I leaned on it. There were days I had to fake it, but soon I realized that I wasn't faking it anymore. I was genuinely happy and felt good about myself again.

One tip I give to help you stay focused is to take progress pictures. At first, this may not sound appealing, but I promise you, as you start to see results, you will wish that you had more pictures to compare your progress with. I sure do! I have my day one pictures, but I waited a month before I took another picture and I wasn't very consistent until a couple of months had gone by. So, even though you may dread those first few pictures, I am encouraging you to take progress pics each week. As your results start to come in, you will soon see in the pictures what you may not be able to see in your mirror, or what you may not hear from the people around you. This will help you to stay focused on your goal and not get discouraged when things get hard.

You have to stay focused, even when you slip. Yep, you're going to have slip ups. Mine came during my second or third month on Keto. Because I am a recovering sugar addict, I had not included any sweets (even keto friendly) into my meal plans (I do currently include some keto friendly sweet treats in my eating plans). I had gone the entire time without anything sweet, but as time went on, I had gotten desperate for something sweet. I followed several Keto groups on social media and had seen several posts talking about how great the sugar-free chocolates from Russel Stover are. I decided one day to stop on my way home to pick some up from my local grocery store. I looked and looked but (of course) they didn't have any. Instead of taking that as a sign that I didn't really need the treats I purchased peanut butter cups from another brand that was all organic everything. I figured that it wouldn't be a big deal if I only ate one. I didn't even wait until I got home, I ripped the package open in the car, and took the first bite. I thought I was in heaven for just a second. I then commenced to devouring that peanut butter cup like a starving man. About 10 minutes later the rumbling in my stomach let me know I'd made a horrible mistake! I'll spare you the details but let's just say that a potty emergency ensued. The point of sharing that short but yet necessary story is to let you know that ALL of us have slips or make decisions to go outside of our eating plans from time to time. Maybe it's to satisfy a craving or to celebrate a special occasion. Either way, it's perfectly normal and OK. Enjoy your treat but don't get stuck there.

When you slip, shake it off! Do not let a slip derail the whole Keto train. Again, none of us got to where we are from one celebratory meal or small treat so let's not let that one thing stop us from getting to where we want to go. If you have a slip, don't beat yourself up and go into a place of self-doubt or negative self-talk. Don't go into an extreme fast or participate in extreme exercise. Just go right back into your normal Keto routine, drink water, eat whole foods according to your macros, move your body (exercise) and trust the process. Do all of these things believing that you can be successful, healthy and whole and knowing that even though you may not see it today, your results are coming!

As your results start coming in, understand that they may not come in the form of a difference on the scale. Your first successful result may be a slimmer looking face, a clearer mind, more energy, or looser fitting clothes. We call those types of victories NSV's or non-scale victories. One of my first NSV's came in the form of my underwear being too big! They were starting to fall down under my clothes! Another NSV that I enjoyed early on was that my back, legs and feet didn't hurt anymore. The pain and inflammation were healed, and I could enjoy going out and doing things that required me to stand and walk again!

No matter what form your successes take, CELEBRATE THEM! Celebrate yourself and do not wait for anyone else to notice. Yes, it would be great if all our friends, family, and our significant other or spouse noticed our first 15-pound weight loss month or our slimmer looking face or waistline, but the truth is that they may not - at first. It doesn't change the fact that it is success and that doesn't make it any less wonderful, so celebrate it!

It's very exciting when you see that your hard work is paying off. I have a little dance that I do when I hit the checkpoints that I set up for myself (it's called the "You Go Girl" dance). I broke my goals down into smaller checkpoints so that I wouldn't have to wait until I made it to my destination to celebrate. Understand that your destination might change along the way, but the point remains the same. You have to celebrate the victories, whether big or small, whether people are celebrating with you or not, and whether it is a scale victory or NSV

Once I got my mind set firm and focused on my success, it was off to the races! Please know that this journey is different for everyone. We all lose at different rates and the changes in our bodies may occur in different areas. When I started, I watched a video from a woman who lost 90 pounds in 6 months! I was so excited to think that I could get in that kind of shape in such a short time but, as it turned out, that was not my story. It has taken me a little longer, and I have not (yet) lost 90 pounds. It's alright because I am so happy with how my story is playing out. Comparison is the thief of happiness, and we all deserve happiness so let's not compare our journey to anyone else's.

At the end of the day, you can read all the books and buy all of the gym clothes and shoes you want, but if you truly don't believe in yourself, the success you're looking for will elude you. I truly believe that is what propelled me through my journey, my all-out belief that my hard work would eventually pay off. I chose to believe in myself again, and that one small thing changed my life.

*If we change our minds, we will change our lives*

# Chapter 2: So...What is Keto Anyway???

The first question that I always get asked, when I tell people that I've lost 80 pounds (to date) in about 7 months through the ketogenic way of eating is, "What is Keto?". I hope to explain in a way that doesn't make me sound like a boring junior high school science teacher.

Keto is the process of retraining the body to move away from using carbohydrates, which in simple terms are sugar molecules - as its main source of fuel. Instead Keto allows us to train our body to use fat as its energy source. Keto is a high (healthy) fat, moderate protein, low carb way of eating. Ketogenic eating is accomplished through the eating of low carb, moderate protein, and high healthy fat diet. I feel compelled to repeat that sentence because it seems counterintuitive for most of us, eating fat will help us get healthy and lose weight, but it's true. By retraining our body to use fat as its main source of energy through reducing our intake of carbohydrates and eating healthy fats to feel satisfied, we burn our body fat! When we're talking about eating keto, 5% of our daily caloric intake should come from carbohydrates. 25% of our daily caloric intake should come from protein. 70% of our daily caloric intake should come from healthy fats.

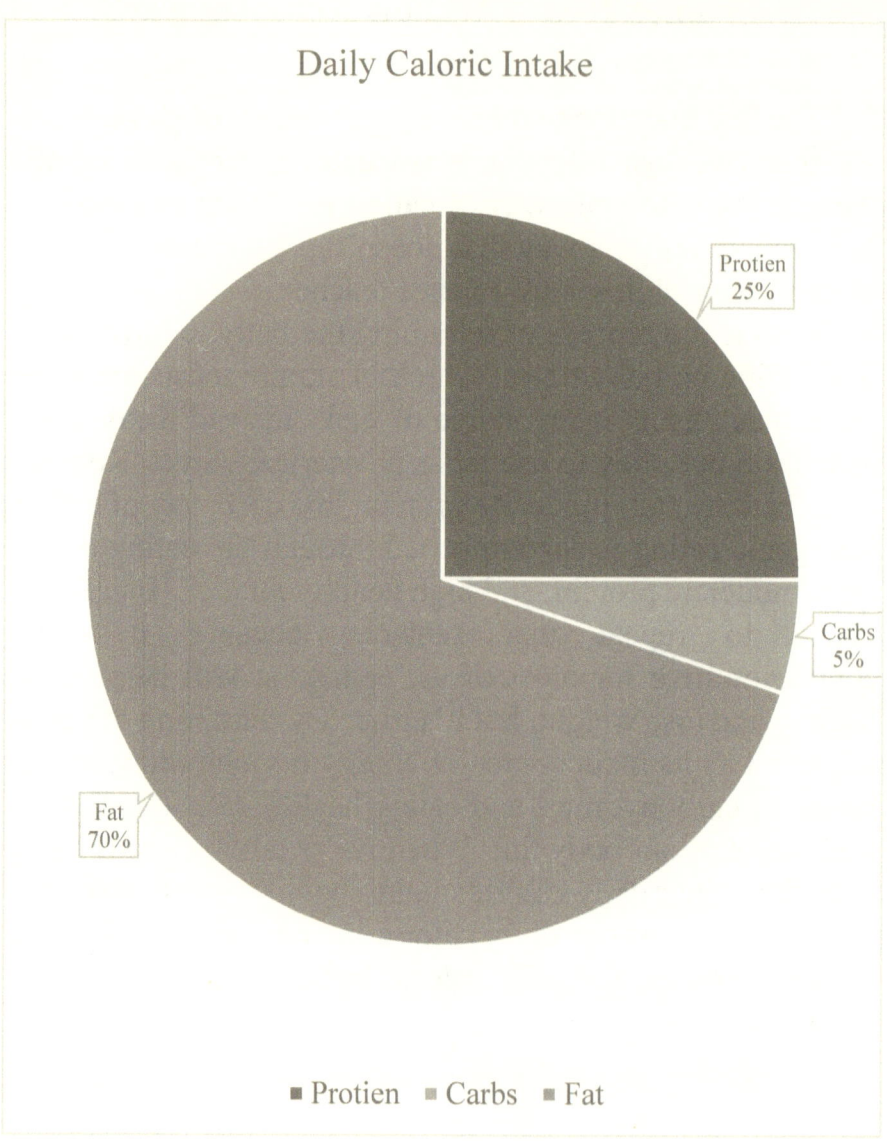

Generally, many of us are eating the Standard American Diet (S.A.D) which consists of us starting our day with a nice bowl of cereal and milk, or maybe a breakfast sandwich and fruit cup from our favorite fast food place, or a donut/muffin and coffee. I loved stopping at the Sonic drive through on my way to work but, what would make my day is if someone brought donuts into the office. I could never resist them, especially if there were apple fritters!

For lunch, we may have a sandwich and chips, or a burger and fries, or even pasta and a salad. For dinner, a meal which for many of us is the biggest meal of the day, it could be any carb and meat dish filled to the brim with pasta, potatoes, bread, and grease. Between each of these meals, there are countless snacking options from pastries, cakes, and pies, to candy and chips…even for the more health conscious one among us, there are sugary and starchy fruits such as watermelon, apples and bananas to eat between meals, when you get sleepy and have that "2:30 feeling" in the middle of the day at work, or just to fill the space when you are bored or lonely. There are countless sweet and salty, crunchy and chewy ways to fill yourself to the brim with carbohydrates that the body can use for energy, and I've probably tried them all

## Here's the Boring Science-y Part

The problem for many of us occurs when we fill ourselves with these carbohydrates, but we don't use all the energy that those calories produce. In simple terms, some of what isn't used get stored in the liver as sort of a energy reserve tank, and the rest gets stored as body fat. In more complex terms, when we eat, our blood sugar rises, which is the signal for our pancreas to produce the hormone insulin to help turn the sugar in our blood (glucose) into energy. That energy gets transported and used to the feed the cells in our body. When everything is functioning like a well-oiled machine, the cells get what they need, and your body uses everything that is put in it, leaving you feeling and looking great. Unfortunately, for most of us, that's not what happens.

Many of us eat way more carbohydrates (sugar) than our bodies need, and as a result, the pancreas produces more insulin to regulate the sugar in the blood. Soon our cells become full and the receptors begin to ignore the signals that the insulin hormones are trying to send out, BUT, because there is still so much sugar in the blood, the pancreas continues to release more insulin. When this happens, it makes it really hard to stabilize the blood sugar. Additionally, it makes it hard for the body to use the fat that gets stored. We begin to store up even more body fat and worse, the fat gets stored around our gut and vital organs. As our pancreas continues to release more insulin constantly, we become Insulin Resistant, which is a precursor to pre-diabetes and metabolic syndrome. Signs and symptoms of pre-diabetes and metabolic syndrome, which occur as a result of insulin resistance, can include things like extreme thirst and frequent urination, skin tags and moles, darkening of the skin in areas such as the armpits, neck, inside of the thighs and groin area (acanthosis nigricans), heart disease, high blood pressure, and of course weight gain. Insulin Resistance is also associated with depression, anxiety and other mood disorders. Furthermore, down the road, if the course of events is allowed to continue, that insulin resistance can develop into full-blown diabetes.

On the other hand, ketosis, the burning of ketones for energy, occurs through the process of ketogenesis. When there is a dramatic reduction in the amount of carbohydrates introduced into the body and the body burns through its reserve stores of glucose, it begins to search for a new energy source. In really simple terms, when you reduce the carbohydrates (sugar) coming into your body to around 5% of your daily caloric intake or about 20 net grams of carbs, your body begins the process of converting body and dietary fat into ketones in the liver, and those ketones are transported to the cells to be used for energy. There are actually three ketone molecules that are produced and used as fuel throughout the body – Acetone, Acetoacetate and Beta-Hydroxybutyrate.

To get into the state of ketosis, you would need to lower the levels of insulin in your body. This can be achieved by eating a diet reduced in carbohydrates and being mindful of the amount of protein consumed as well as fasting for some time. The state of ketosis is completely natural but, achieving it can be very individualized. For most people, the rule of thumb is to reduce the carbohydrate intake to down to around 20 (net) grams per day. However, there are some people out there that can eat up to 50 (net) grams of carbs per day and remain in ketosis. It really just depends on your individual body.

# Health Benefits of Ketosis

Being in the state of ketosis provides the body with so many health benefits. The first advantage is that ketones are a "clean" source of energy for the brain. The brain uses about 20% of the body's energy - more than any other organ in the body to keep it running. When using glucose as their main energy source, many people find themselves in a fog, very tired, and unable to concentrate during times when they haven't refueled with carbs and sugar. I know in my own experience, prior to starting the keto way of eating, I had such a brain fog that it almost seemed that I could not access important information when I needed it most. I was always tired, cranky, and had a very difficult time focusing on small details. However, on ketones, many feel a mental clarity they've never experienced previously, and for me, the difference was like night and day. Information that I struggled to access or memories that I struggled to recall seemed to be front and center in my mind. It seemed that my decision-making ability was sharpened, and my overall cognitive function just felt clear and effortless. Think of the difference between a machine that runs of coal (glucose) versus one that runs on solar power (fat). That is the difference between using glucose and fat as the body and brain's main source of energy. Glucose is not very efficient, and there is that seemingly constant need to keep resupplying more whereas most people have much more fat stored up in the body than sugar. This means there is a constant supply of energy...no more 2:30 feeling!

Other health benefits of ketosis include the reversal of conditions such as insulin resistance, metabolic syndrome, pre-diabetes, and type 2 diabetes. Keto was used for many years to control epileptic seizures in children and has shown promise in helping people suffering from PCOS (polycystic ovary syndrome) and certain types of cancers. Additionally, other benefits such as the improvement of rheumatoid arthritis, joint pain, inflammation, acne, the reduction of migraines, increases in physical endurance and (of course!) **WEIGHT LOSS** is also experienced by people who practice the ketogenic way of eating and, let's face it, this is what a few of us are here for. So then, the question becomes, how do we get started? Well... I'm glad you asked!

Verizon LTE
11:41 AM
July 29
2:50 PM
Edit

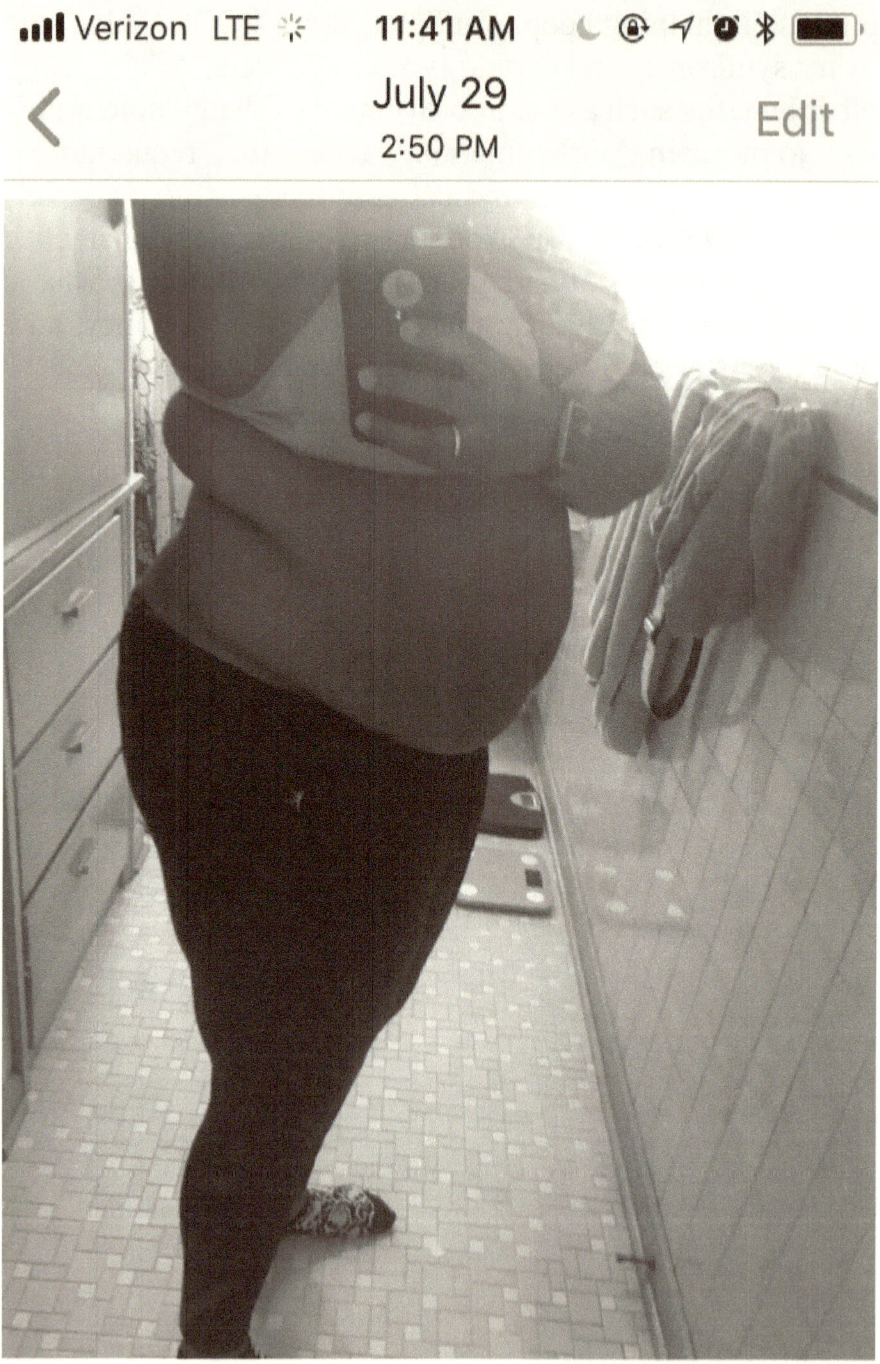

# Chapter 3: How Do We Get Started on Keto?

## Step 1: So, You Want to Start Keto? Time to Get Your Research On

I started keto on July 28th, 2018. There were no bells and whistles that day, and I didn't initially believe that the day was a particularly special day. Little did I know it would be like a second birthday for me! I'd been sitting in my office at home, scrolling through social media and clicking through about a ton of open webpages. I had finally become so sick of being sick and tired that for about a week I'd read through what felt like millions of websites and watched hours of videos on YouTube, all to get a handle on this thing called Keto. Before I set out on my research, the only thing I've ever heard about Keto was how it must be unhealthy because it excludes fruit and "you know you can't be healthy without fruit!". When I think back to how I almost let one person's (false) opinion about Keto keep me from experiencing all the health benefits and weight loss success I've experienced so far, I almost laugh!

**The second piece of sisterly advice is to do your own research!**

Do not let the opinions of others, who may or may not be informed, be the deciding factor on your health decisions. When going through the process of conducting your research on Keto, or any other way of eating, make sure that you are considering all sides, not just the one that you want to be "right." It seems like common sense but, listen to both sides of the argument. Take down notes and read them over during the process of deciding whether this way of eating is right for you or not.

Another factor that needs to be a part of your decision-making process should be to take an honest evaluation of your health, as it stands today – not what you think it is, not what it used to be, and not what you wish it is, but a brutally honest evaluation of exactly where you stand today. This will also include making a visit to your doctor's office to discuss the state of your affairs and how Keto could be used to improve things for you. Understand this: Although there is a lot of evidence that points to the benefits of Keto there are still many doctors, nurses, nutritionists, and other health care professionals that are staunchly against their patients practicing this way of eating and there are many reasons for this. I am extremely lucky that my health care provider was very pleased when I informed him that I was changing my lifestyle to incorporate Keto. He had implored me to "stop eating carbs" as he was explaining my pre-diabetic diagnosis, so he was pretty thrilled at the conclusion that I had come to.

As I have previously stated at the beginning of this book, I am not a medical doctor or provider. I have the utmost respect for the work that medical professionals provide. This book is in no way to be used as a tool to diagnose any condition or should it be used to cure any disease processes. However, if you do not have an explainable condition that is counter indicated for Keto, and your doctor can only give you his or her opinion of what they think Keto is, you may want to find another provider that will be more supportive of your decision to improve your health through making better nutritional decisions.

As you are conducting your research and making an honest assessment of your situation, you would do well to write everything down. Get a notebook specifically to document your Keto journey. Make a list of the websites and studies that you found helpful and informative so that you can refer to them while speaking with your doctor. Take notes on the things your doctor has to say as well. As I was watching YouTube videos from Dr. Eric Berg and Thomas DeLauer (my two personal FAVORITE resources for Keto information), I took notes so that I could refer to them as I was making my plan on how I was going to implement Keto in my life, which brings me to my third piece of sisterly advice.

**The third piece of sisterly advice is to make a plan and WRITE IT DOWN.**

### Step 2: Build Your Action Plan

On the flip side of that coin, there is a lot of evidence out there that suggests that there are some people that will essentially plan themselves to death and never actually start anything because they don't have their plan together, it's called analysis paralysis. Anyone that follows My Sister's Keto on social media knows that I am a big advocate for not only planning but for starting as well. I believe that there must be a happy balance between making a plan and going through the processes of actually executing the work of that plan to achieve your goals and dreams.

The truth is that 70% of people who start a plan, quit. However, people who make a plan and then **write it down** are over 40% more likely to carry it out through fruition! Let's be real here, weight loss, as we know it, is hard enough, if writing down your plan on how you were going to make healthy changes in your life gave you a 40% advantage over not doing it, why would anyone not? By writing down your plans, it allows you to see the clear action steps that you will take to become successful, this will keep you on track. It also provides you with motivation for the days when you don't think you can keep going. In fact, by keeping a detailed journal of your entire process, you can easily see where you started and how far you've come. One thing to know is this: **you DO NOT have to have your plan completely fleshed out to start**. Treat your action plan as a living document, meaning that as you go along your journey, there will be somethings that need to be added, adjusted, or taken out of the plan. It is not written in stone.

### So, What Should Be in Your Action Plan?

Your action plan can be as simple or complicated as you make it, but it is my recommendation that you keep track of the following information:

1. The date you started.

2. Your age and your height.

3. Your starting weight, body fat percentage, and BMR

   (there are online calculators to get this information).

4. Measurements of your neck, arms, legs, bust, waist,

   and hips.

5. Any medical conditions you have been diagnosed

   with.

6. A list of any medications you are taking and their dosages.

7. Your goal weight.

Once you have your starting stats recorded, on the next page, you will start to record how you plan to accomplish your goals through Keto. When I say write everything down in your plan, I mean that you should be planning out and writing down what time you plan to eat your meals, how much water you plan to consume and by what time, What time you plan to take your vitamins, etc. The more detailed your plan, the better off you will be. Keep two things in mind, I said detailed NOT complicated! This is simply a plan, and it will be your guide to help you remember to do things and to track your progress. If you don't execute it perfectly the first few times, don't beat yourself up. Just look at what you *are* doing and when you're doing it and decide whether the plan needs to be adjusted. At the end of the day, you know your success is on its way! All you have to do is make it happen, and your plan is your guide to doing just that.

### Figuring Out Your Macros

One of the first steps to planning your path to Keto success is figuring out what your macronutrients should be. As we previously stated, Ketogenic eating is accomplished through the eating of a low carb, moderate protein, and high healthy fat diet. About 5% of your daily caloric intake should come from carbohydrates, 25% of your daily caloric intake should come from protein and 70% of your daily calories should come from healthy fats. But what does that look like for you? Well, figuring out (and tracking) your macros is not as hard as it may seem. Most people simply go online and find a Keto macros counter/tracker. There are several options out there that will meet that need such as Carb Manager, My Fitness Pal, If It Fits Your Macros, Ruled.Me, and others. The example pictures that are in this book come from Carb Manager. It is a free application for your smartphone (both iOS and Android), there is also a desktop webpage as well; however, remember, there are plenty of other options out there so, you do not have to use this one.

Most macro counters are very easy to set up. Many will want you to input your sex, age, height, weight, and level of activity. In some cases, it may ask you for your body fat percentage. If you don't have a smart scale or other means to get that information, many times the macro counter site will supply pictures and ask you to select the one that is closest to representing your body. You plug in the information, and the app will supply you with your base calories (what you need to maintain your current state). At that point, you will input your weekly weight loss goal. Keep in mind: It takes a deficit of about 3500 calories to burn 1 pound of body fat. The app will usually automatically reduce the daily caloric goals then calculate your daily macronutrients from there.

**Example**: A 42-year-old woman, 5 foot 8 inches tall, weighing in at 210 lbs, and leads a sedentary life decides she wants to lose 1.5 pounds a week. She inputs her information into the Carb Manager app, and it tells her that if she desired no changes to her weight, her daily caloric goal would be about 2284 calories per day. However, she wants to lose around 1.5 pounds a week or about 6 pounds in a month, through caloric deficit. The app subtracts the appropriate number of calories from her original base calories to supply her with her new daily caloric goal of 1576 calories per day. In the next step, the app will then tell her what her macronutrient breakdown will be for each day.

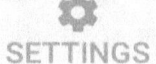 SETTINGS

 **MY PROFILE**

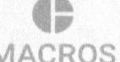 MACROS

 DIET

ⓘ We'll use this info to help determine your diet & health goals and to analyze your progress.

## My Profile

Gender:
Female ▾

Year of Birth:
1977 ▾

Height:
5 feet ▾    8 inches ▾

Need Help?

SETTINGS

MY PROFILE

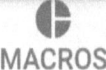
**MACROS**

DIET

## Macros Calculator

Let's start by setting a **calories goal** based on whether your want to lose weight, maintain, or build muscle. Select how much you want to decrease or increase your calories.

Need Help?

**Lose Weight**: -31% Calories Deficit

Calories Goal

1576

At this calories goal, we predict that you will lose 6.1 lbs per month.

Next, let's calculate your

Carbs : Protein : Fat Ratio

**5:25:70 (Keto)** ▾

5% Net Carbs: **20**     g

25% Protein: **99**     g

70% Fat: **123**     g

**APPLY MY MACROS**    Everyday ▾

Advanced ⌄

Need Help?

Now that you have your daily calorie goals, the app then breaks it down even further into the allotted grams for each macronutrient. In the case of our example, supposing she sticks to the 70:25:5 ketogenic protocol, her 5% daily allowance of carbs would be 20 (net) grams, her 25% of protein equates to about 99 grams and 70% daily allowance of fat would be 123 grams of fat. These macronutrients are the building blocks of your daily diet. Once you have that information, you can begin to plan out your meals, your grocery shopping list, and begin to execute your plan for wellness, health, and weight loss.

One other thing I'd like to point out before I close this chapter. In this book, when I talk about carbs, I am expressing that amount in net grams. Net grams are total carbohydrate grams minus grams of fiber and sugar alcohols such as xylitol and erythritol. So, if an item has a total carb count of 10 grams but has 5 grams of fiber and 1 gram of sugar alcohols, the net carb total would be 4. That would be the number that you track in your counter. In the example on the next page, our item has a total carb count of 10 grams and a fiber count of 5 grams, leaving us with 5 net grams of carbohydrates. Of course, you could track total carbs; however, for the sake of this book, I am solely referencing net grams.

# Nutrition Facts

Serving size

**Amount Per Serving**

## Calories

# 0

% Daily Value*

| | |
|---|---|
| **Total Fat** 5g | **6%** |
| Saturated Fat 0g | **0%** |
| *Trans* Fat 0g | |
| **Sodium** 0mg | **0%** |
| **Total Carbohydrate** 10g | **4%** |
| Dietary Fiber 5g | **18%** |
| Total Sugars 0g | |
| Includes 0g Added Sugars | **0%** |
| **Protein** 5g | **10%** |

Not a significant source of cholesterol, vitamin D, calcium, iron, and potassium

*The % Daily Value (DV) tells you how much a nutrient in a serving of food contributes to a daily diet. 2,000 calories a

# Chapter 4: What Do We Eat on Keto?

## Step 4: Make a list and Check it Twice

Now that you know what your macros look like, you have to figure out what to eat to achieve those numbers. It's pretty easy to figure out what you'll want to avoid while enjoying the keto way of eating (starchy vegetables and fruits, bread pastas, rice, beans, potatoes, sugar, sugary snacks, and most processed foods. If it comes from a box, you probably shouldn't eat it). You want to stick with the outside walls of your grocery store, and, for the most part, stick with whole foods to meet your needs. It seems easy, but when you visit any social media Keto group, you will see the question being asked all over the place, 'What can we eat' or 'Is this Keto?', Which leads me to my next piece of advice

## The fourth piece of sisterly advice is KISS (Keep It Simple, Sis)

Look, I know how easy it can be to get caught up in trying new recipes or trying to keep our taste buds engaged and happy, while also starting a new way of eating. BUT it will be much easier for you to start your Keto journey and maintain it if you keep your meals simple. You will save money on your grocery bill as well. I have made the mistake of spending countless dollars on expensive ingredients to create a dish that I saw online only to taste it and hate it!

What do I mean by keeping it simple? You should start by choosing to make meals that are so simple that even your family members that don't eat "Keto" can enjoy. It will save you time, money, and make it easy for you to track your macros in the beginning. Simply choose a good source of protein, your favorite low carb green leafy vegetable, and a fat source that will allow you to be satiated until your next meal. Keep in mind that although the caloric protocol for keto is 70:25:5, these numbers represent caloric intake, **not** the actual amount of food that is sitting on your plate. When you're looking at your plate of food, it should resemble the second pie chart on the next page. Although your daily caloric intake of carbs should be about 5% (around 20 net grams per day), you should be aiming to eat between 5-7 cups of veggies. This means that most of your plate should be filled with vegetables. Items like spinach, salad greens, cucumbers, and broccoli, while they are high in nutrients, they are also very low calorie, so you can eat a higher volume and not bust your macros whereas fat is much more calorically dense per volume, so you won't have to eat much fat to get in the necessary grams.

# Macros

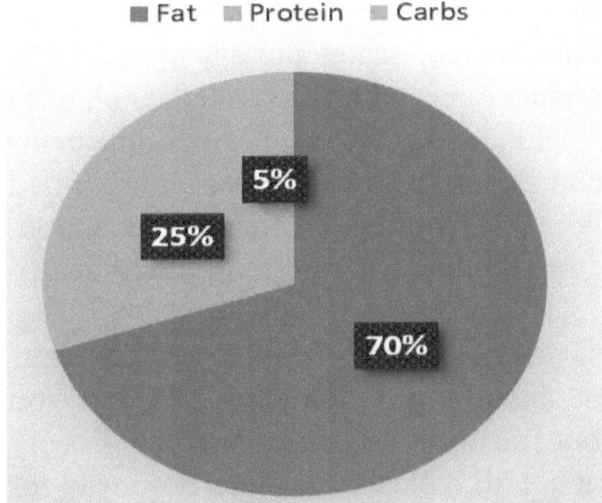

What Your Plate Should look Like

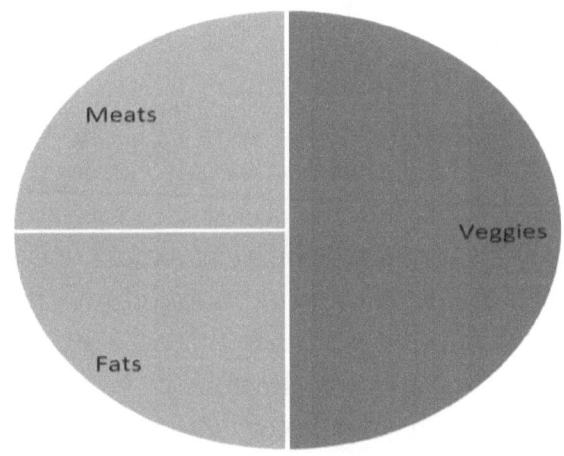

At the beginning of my journey, most of which I have documented on the My Sister's Keto Diet Instagram page, I kept my meals extremely simple. I ate dishes such as keto taco salad and chili (no beans), bacon and eggs, steak with veggies, bun-less cheese burgers with a side salad, or chicken and avocado salad. I loaded up on veggies making items such as zucchini noodles, mashed cauliflower, and stuffed bell peppers. As I got more confident, comfortable, and fat adapted, I began to try out different and more complicated recipes.

In the following sections, I am including a list of items to help get your thoughts going on the types of foods you could use to plan your meals and pick up from the grocery store. These lists are not all inclusive as there is no way for me to know exactly what each of you like or desire to eat.

## Protein

Protein is vital for building and repairing tissue, blood, bones, hormones and other chemical processes in the body. If you don't get enough protein, these processes can start to be compromise and break down the lean muscle in the body; however, for many of us, protein is the heart of a meal. Most people need to ensure that they're getting enough and that can be accomplished by simply measuring food portions. Remember, in terms of your macros, Protein is your goal macro. It is the one you want to meet every day.

You'll want to stick with pasture-fed and grass-fed options, if you can afford them. While it is a little more expensive, you'll avoid eating meats that were exposed to antibiotics and hormones. Don't worry if you can't afford to pay the extra costs for it. You will be able to maintain keto whether you eat grass-fed meats or not. You just want to buy the best quality foods you can afford. When picking the protein source for your meals, for instance, ground beef, you don't want to pick the leanest, 95/5, but something a little fattier like 85/15 instead.

Good sources of protein include the following:

**Beef:** Steaks, Roast, Ground Beef, Ribs

**Poultry**: Chicken, Turkey

**Eggs**

**Pork:** Chops, Tenderloins, Ham (watch for brown sugar cured)

**Lamb**

**Fish:** Salmon, Tuna, Cod, Mahi Mahi Sardines

**Seafood:** Crabs, Shrimp, Lobster, Mussels

**Organ Meat**: Heart, Liver, Tongue

**Cold Cuts:** be cautious with these because many contain sugars and other flavorings

**Nuts and seeds**: considered a source of protein and fat but be careful when consuming. They often contain carbs and are a higher calorie food. It is really easy to overeat these items if you don't have portions measured out beforehand.

**Full Fat Dairy:** a source of protein and fat but use with caution as some people experience inflammation and a weight loss stall with overconsumption

## Carbohydrates

While enjoying the Keto lifestyle we know that up to 5% of your daily caloric intake should come from carbohydrates. The lower your carb intake, the more your body is forced to use ketones for energy. That's where the magic happens, folks! Most people get wrapped up in where these carbs come from. Instead of eating the sugary simple carbs that come with most processed foods, table sugar, and sugary fruits, you want to replace those things with green leafy and non-starchy vegetables. The goal with your vegetables is to get 5-7 cups daily. Other Keto friendly carbs include dairy, natural cheeses, nuts (which are also a source of protein and contain fat as well), seeds, and berries. Yes, there are some fruits that you can enjoy!

Good sources of carbohydrates include the following:

Spinach
Cauliflower
Kale
Bell peppers
Zucchini
Broccoli
Mushrooms
Full fat dairy products (milk, cheeses, heavy whipping cream etc.)
Bok choy
Jicama
Onions and garlic
Cucumbers
Asparagus
Cabbage
Collard Greens
Radishes
Brussel sprouts
Eggplant
Berries (Blueberries, Raspberries, Strawberries) – enjoy in limited amounts.

# Fats

Although everywhere you look in the keto community we're talking about how this way of eating is a higher fat lifestyle, do not get it twisted. This is not a fat for the sake of eating fat free for all. When I am speaking about fat in this book, and to my clients, I am talking about high healthy fats. As I previously mentioned, fat is what keeps you from wanting to eat your desk in the middle of the day when your coworkers are enjoying their second pizza party in a week! It keeps you satiated and full of energy. For most people, once they become fat adapted and are feeling more comfortable with this way of eating, they reduce the amount of dietary fat that they are eating and let their bodies turn into a bodyfat burning machine! This process happens at different rates for everyone so be patient with yourself.

Good Sources of healthy fats include the following:

Avocado
Avocado Oil
Beef Tallow
Butter (NOT Margarine)
Natural Cheeses
Cream Cheese
Heavy Whipping Cream
Coconut Oil
Extra Virgin Olive Oil
Ghee
MCT Oil
Mayonnaise (beware of hidden sugars and canola and soybean oils)

Olives

Bacon Fat, Lard, Duck Fat

As already mentioned in the list, avoid getting your fats from sources such as canola oil, corn oil, grapeseed oil, peanut oil, safflower oil, and soybean oil, as many of these could contain trans-fats and/or Omega 6 fatty acids. Eating too much of these can result in the increased risk of blood clots, inflammation issues and increased risk of heart disease.

## Sweeteners

When I first began my keto journey, one of the first things I cut out of my diet was sugar, and it was by far the hardest thing in my life to cut. I am a recovering sugar addict, and there is sugar in everything! Did you know that the average American consumes over 1 ½ cups of sugar daily? Back in our Grandparents day that was unheard of! I had no real idea of how much sugar had been implanted into just about everything, until I started keto and really started to read labels and do the legwork. Sugar is an ingredient in most processed foods, there is added sugar in most sauces, seasoning, and there is even sugar in products such as cough and allergy medications.

If you truly want to be effective in your keto experience, you have to be diligent about reading food labels and ingredients lists before you purchase a product and get it home. When it comes to sugar while enjoying the ketogenic lifestyle, it is advisable to avoid it as well as artificial sweeteners. They will raise the levels of sugar (glucose) in the blood, inducing an insulin response in the body, which will kick you out of ketosis.

Here is a short list of sweeteners that are **NOT** Keto friendly and should be avoided

Table Sugar
Coconut Sugar
Brown Sugar
Honey
Agave
Maple Syrup
High Fructose Corn Syrup
Splenda
Maltodextrin
Maltitol
Maltose
Aspartame
Sucrose

Here is a list of sweeteners that **ARE** Keto **FRIENDLY** and can be used in dishes and drinks
Stevia
Erythritol
Monk Fruit
Swerve
*Xylitol
*Xylitol can cause stomach upset even when consumed in small amounts. In increased quantities such as those used in baking, Xylitol has been shown to kick some people out of ketosis. Use caution when deciding to use this product.

Be careful and read labels when selecting sweeteners from the grocery store as some manufacturers are trying to cash in on our Keto curiosity. Some products claim to be Stevia or Monk Fruit but also contain sugar or other bulking agents that can keep you from reaching ketosis or knock you out of ketosis.

## Other Products

The following is a list of other items that aren't mandatory to start Keto however they may be helpful as a substitution when making some of your favorite dishes align with your new Keto lifestyle:

Almond Flour
Coconut Flour
Pork Rinds
Xanthan Gum
Coconut Aminos
Flavored Extracts
Collagen Powder
Cocoa Powder
Catsup and BBQ Sauce Sweetened with Stevia
Protein Powder

Now that you have an idea of the types of foods that you like, that are also Keto friendly, and have begun thinking up the delicious dishes you can make with these ingredients, my next piece of sisterly advice is to make your food decisions ahead of time and put it in your plan.

**The fifth piece of sisterly advice is to make a grocery list that spells out your plan for each meal of the week.**

The reason for this advice is simple. If you write your list out by the meal, you will not forget anything, and you will not feel compelled to purchase outside of your planned meals. Trust me, while it may cost you a few extra minutes, it will save you at the cash register.

**Step 5: Now that you've got all of your healthy foods purchased and put away, it's time to START**
**The sixth piece of sisterly advice is just DO IT.**

You've already made the commitment and investment by doing your research and buying your groceries. You've made your meal plan, so what could possibly stop you? Well, here are a couple of issues I've experienced that might have stopped me in my journey had I not gotten my mind set on my success very early in the process.

***Issue #1 Believing that it's too complicated or "too much work to count macros"***: Earlier, in chapter 3, we talked about setting up your macro counter/tracker (ex. Carb Manager or My Fitness Pal). These free or low-cost tools make it easy to keep your food intake and macros logged in one easy to find place. Other tools that will help you immensely along your journey are a food scale, measuring cups, and measuring spoons. These items will allow you to accurately know (and therefore track) your portion sizes. This is important because it is very hard, especially in the beginning, to trust your eyes when it comes to eyeballing or guessing portion sizes and those macros/calories do matter. No matter what way of eating you choose, whether it's Keto or not, you need to be in a caloric deficit in order to lose weight. I am not saying that you will have to measure and/or track your foods forever. In fact, I stopped measuring and tracking a few months into my journey and even now as I am writing this book, I've currently lost 81 pounds and continue to lose. By starting these processes in the beginning, you will set yourself up for success.

Yes, you can totally start keto and lose weight without tracking macros and weighing/measuring food portions. BUT, if you are keeping up with portion sizes, you have better control of what you're taking in without the unexpected overeating of calories or undereating. Also, by keeping a more accurate log, it allows you to go back and examine how your body is reacting to your new lifestyle and the foods you eat. This is especially important if you find yourself experiencing a weight loss stall or (worse yet) weight gain! This happened to me. I was measuring and tracking most of my foods…just not the butter that I was using. Anytime I used butter, which was several times in my meals, I would just use the little lines on the side of the package. One week, during my weigh in, I noticed that my weight had not moved and the next week I gained! As I started to go through my log, I really couldn't figure out what I needed to tighten up on. I wasn't eating sweeteners at the time and my dairy consumption was pretty low (those are common reasons that a lot of people stall) so I decided to get a little tighter on my measuring and weighing and behold… I found the issue! It turns out that those little lines on the butter package are misleading (surprise surprise). I was actually eating TWICE what I thought that I was, and let me tell you, when you use butter several times a day it can really (REALLY) add up! If a tablespoon of butter is 100 calories and you think you're using two or three tablespoons a day, but it turns out you're using four to six…that's 400 to 600 calories of just butter a day! Not good.

Just do yourself a favor, even if it's only for the first couple of weeks – measure, weigh and track. You can thank me later!

*Issue #2: Having non-keto friendly foods/snacks available, especially when you don't have anything to do around the house.* This one is super common, especially when you have family members and kids that don't keep Keto. A part of the solution to this issue is just plain old self-discipline. I know this isn't sexy or fun, but there is no other way around it. This is why getting your mind settled in the beginning is so important. You have to exercise your will to know that you don't *really* want to eat junk food. You want your body to become effective at burning your bodyfat for energy and the only way to get there is to cut the carbs, sugar, and processed foods. Trust me, Little Debbie and I used to roll tight together, especially when I was home on the weekends, watching television or spending idle time scrolling on social media. I wish I could say it was just me and old Debbie, but the truth is Betty Crooker used to be right with us. We were a whole clique with Sara Lee riding shotgun.

At the end of the day, the truth is that when I changed my way of eating, other parts of my life changed as well. As my waistline shrank, my confidence began to grow, and I found myself going back out into the world again, traveling for work and leisure. I was no longer afraid to be more active. I don't worry anymore about the pain in my back, feet or my legs stopping me from being physically active. Being out and about also kept me from doing the boredom eating that keeps a lot of us stuck.

*Issue #3: Having to cook for non-keto eaters:* I also had this problem as well, though maybe not to the severity as some people with young children might experience. I am the mother of two very independent teenaged girls, so when I first started my keto journey, I would cook dinner for my family only a few nights a week, and I certainly was not cooking three times a day, seven days a week. My husband and daughters do their fair share of the family meal preparation. On the days I cooked for them, it was challenging because I would try everything possible to manage my own meal tracking and preparation while trying to cook their food, without tasting it. Another thing I struggled with was snacking as I cooked, which is something I still work on some days. It used to be nothing to have a glass (or two) of wine and take a taste here and there while I was cooking, but once I started Keto, it was a whole paradigm shift that I continue to work through. Now instead of wine and bread, I may instead pop a couple of olives in my mouth if I'm hungry while I'm cooking.

**To avoid a whole mess and being tempted to snack while cooking a separate meal for your family, my advice is to try to make your meal first or meal prep ahead of time.**
If you already have your meal planned out and put into your macro counter, cook your meal first. Some people actually cook a few days' worth of meals ahead of time to save even more time! If you can swing it, you will not have to try and do all the tracking, measuring and weighing while you are hungry and trying to prepare food for your family and yourself. Doing all of that while you are hungry is setting yourself up to fail because your temptation to snack will be hard to resist.

When deciding what you're going to make for dinner (or whichever meal you choose), it will help you a LOT to choose meals that can easily be enjoyed by everyone in the house whether are Keto or not. Not only is this a time saver but it is also a money saver as well. Here are some examples of keto meals that the entire family can enjoy:

# Breakfast

Bacon and Eggs
Crustless Quiche
Keto Pancakes
Breakfast Chia Pudding
Keto Oatmeal
Omelets
Breakfast pizza
Bulletproof coffee

## Lunch

Tuna Salad with dill relish and mayonnaise
Bunless cheeseburgers or other sandwich
Chopped Salad with full-fat Salad Dressing
Ham and Cheese Rolls
Cabbage rolls.
Lettuce Wraps

## Dinner

Taco salad (no shell, beware of store-bought taco seasoning, it may contain sneaky sugar)
Bunless cheese burgers
Baked chicken with veggies
Spaghetti with meat sauce (you get Shirataki noodles; your family gets regular spaghetti Choose sauce that has no added sugar and watch your portion size)
Chicken Alfredo (with homemade sauce and zucchini noodles)
Steak and/or shrimp with veggies
Stuffed green peppers

Again, these meals are really simple, they don't take a lot of complicated or expensive ingredients, and they also don't take a lot of time to prepare. For many of us weighing and tracking will be time consuming enough, so you'll want to make it as easy as you can on yourself in the beginning.

## Drink Water

This should really go without saying, but as we are going along on this keto journey, it is imperative that you are drinking the appropriate amount of water for you. There are some schools of thought that say that eight 8oz glasses of water per day is an appropriate amount. Other say that you should be drinking at least half (1/2) of your body weight in ounces of water. There are still others that say that you should be drinking one full gallon of water per day. It is my belief that you should be somewhere in between the parameters of those three schools of thought. If you are getting between 64oz and 128oz of water, you're on the right track. I would say that to get the absolute best results water is your best bet for a thirst quencher.

There are some that absolutely can't stand the taste of water but, it is my opinion that you will want to avoid drinking diet sodas that are filled with artificial sweeteners, which have been associated with health concerns such as increased risk of heart disease and certain cancers. There are keto friendly soft drinks available that do not contain artificial sweeteners. Additionally, you can enjoy natural teas and coffee sweetened with keto friendly sweeteners as well.

# Chapter 6: Weight Loss

**The seventh piece of sisterly advice is to not get too caught up on what the scale is (or isn't) doing.**

As we begin the process of cleaning our diet of all the sugar, processed foods and cutting our carb consumption down to around 20 net grams per day, many of us will start to see and feel the changes taking place in our bodies. It seemed that almost immediately the fog that seemed to stop my brain from functioning properly cleared. I was able to think and perform up to my standard again, in fact shortly after beginning my keto life, I interviewed and got a new job after several failed interviews for months prior! In my first week of eating ketogenically, I managed to lose 8 pounds. Then by the end of the first month, I'd lost 14 pounds and I was ecstatic. As happy as I was, there was a hidden part of the process that I didn't know about until I went through it, it was the release of water weight.

Because you are reducing your carbs so drastically, there will be a decline in the insulin response produced in your body, and as you have (hopefully) increased your water consumption, your body begins to flush out water, sodium, and other electrolytes. This is why many of us on keto have such drastic changes so early on in our experience. We lose a lot of water weight and have a noticeable marked decrease in inflammation in our bodies. One thing that I noticed, in my experience, is that almost immediately, I could see the changes in my face from week to week, especially when I look at old photos. My cheeks, eyes, and chin were less puffy, and soon other parts of my body were beginning to be less puffy as well. It seems like there could be no downside to losing that water weight...but there is. It's the dreaded Keto Flu.

## Keto Flu

I decided to give this issue its own little section because everyone has heard of the dreaded keto flu. If you haven't heard of it, once you start keto and join some of the social media groups, you will. Many of us that are living the Keto lifestyle learned about it the hard way, but I'm hoping I can save you the trouble.

The Keto flu is the result of you reducing your carbohydrate intake down to approximately 20 net grams or less per day. This forces your body to convert fat into ketones, which is exactly what you want. However, your body is like a small child who had their sweet candy taken away and so it begins to throw a proverbial fit. It wants the carbs that you have taken away.

As I previously explained, when you start to transition over, and your insulin levels start to drop, your body will react by excreting sodium and other electrolytes in your urine and you will have to urinate A LOT. That's when you start to see the good result of the reduction of some of the inflammation as your body starts to shed the water weight. BUT, before you put on that party hat, there is a downside to losing all of that water and the associated electrolytes. When you have that rapid loss of sodium and other electrolytes, it can cause symptoms such as:

Fatigue
Nausea
Muscle Cramps
Dizziness

Irritability

Headache

In a nutshell, the Keto Flu can make you feel like you have the actual flu. The good news is that it is temporary; many people that get it only feel bad for a couple of days, which was my experience. If you take the advice below, you can either avoid it altogether or only have to suffer for a very short time.

**The eighth piece of sisterly advice is Do Not Let This Stop You!**

The fix for the Keto flu is simple. Since the main cause of the symptoms is the loss of water and sodium, replacing that water and sodium will fix you right up. I recommend having a glass of water first thing in the morning, as soon as you get up. In that glass of water, sprinkle a little bit of pink salt (or whatever salt you have on hand) into the glass and drink it. Then Keep drinking water throughout the day. For most people, drinking ½ of their body weight in ounces of water will keep them plenty hydrated throughout the day. Some people also drink a little bone broth or chicken broth as an alternative to the salt water. Either way, replacing the sodium lost through urination is a very quick way to speed up your keto flu recovery and on your way to fat loss.

If you are experiencing muscle cramps or Charlie horses, especially at night, this can be the result of a magnesium deficiency. An easy fix for this is to eat foods rich in magnesium such as spinach, kale and avocado. Taking a magnesium supplement before bedtime also helps as magnesium is a natural muscle relaxer.

If, for some reason, you are still experiencing symptoms of the keto flu after trying the above remedies - if you are still working out during this time, you may need to lighten up your physical activities until you're feeling better. Also, you may need to slightly increase your carb intake until you're feeling better. Then slowly lower them back down to the recommended 5% (about 20g). If none of these things work, a discussion with your doctor or health care provider may be needed to assess whether this way of eating is for you.

After a bout with keto flu, many of us are on our way in our weight loss journeys. First, many of us may lose a lot of scale weight, but we also notice the changes in our body compositions over time as well. Even for those of us who do not lose any scale weight, rest assured, changes are taking place. For all of us enjoying the Keto lifestyle, there is some internal healing of disease processes in the body that take time to resolve. The body must heal internally for us to really reap the external benefits of this way of eating. Many of us are suffering from medical issues that we may not even know that we have because they went undiagnosed. With that said, be patient with yourself as you are in this early stage of your journey.

Remember that while you may not see a difference on the scale, there may be body composition improvements taking place. Over the course of a few weeks your clothes and shoes may start running a little big. Areas of our bodies that used to be in constant pain are no longer bothering us due to a reduction in inflammation. For some, our skin is clearer than it has been in years. These are the non-scale victories that I was referencing in the beginning of the book. This is why it is important to not just take note of your starting weight but also to also take those body measurements as well. This way you can track those body composition changes instead of beating yourself up over what the scale is saying.

## What if You're Just Not Losing Weight on Keto?

There are a few of us that will have a difficult time losing weight on the scale. Now, while the non-scale victories and inches off of our waistline are nice, we all want the scale to move (down). I know that it can be frustrating and sometimes heartbreaking when you see story after story about another person's success and it not be realized in your scale experience. First, before we get into all the reasons why you may not be losing weight, I want to tell you that comparison is the thief of joy. Please, DO NOT COMPARE YOUR JOURNEY TO ANYBODY ELSE'S. Your success is on its way, but it is not going to happen when your mind is someplace else. It's fine to have goals, but you really want to concentrate on your own journey. With that being said, here are some reasons why the scale might not be moving and what you can do to get it going.

*Issue #1 You may not be in ketosis:* This is a common rookie mistake that can occur when you're eating a lot of keto branded, processed (boxed) food products or too many other hidden carbs such as too much dairy or nuts. Another reason this may be happening is trying to make too many of the pretty keto desserts and treats. One way to prevent this is to track your food intake (including portion sizes) and macros.

The only way to know whether you are truly in ketosis is to test your ketone levels. You can test your ketones either through urine testing (least expensive), breath testing (moderately expensive), or blood testing (most expensive but also most accurate).

*Issue #2 You're eating too much fat:* Yes, Keto is high fat, moderate protein, low carb way of eating but the point of cutting the carbs is to burn body fat, not the dietary fat that you eat. Fats generally tend to have twice the calorie count of protein or carbs so if you're overdoing it on the fats, then you're probably blowing your calories for the day. Overeating by just 500 calories a day every day for a week can result in a one-pound weight gain at the end of the week and even if you didn't eat that way every day, at the very least, you will stall your progress.

*Issue 3 You're not eating enough calories:* On the flip side of eating too many calories is not getting enough. This is super common – I did struggle with this myself. Yes, you want to be in a caloric deficit to lose weight BUT by going too low, you risk your metabolism slowing to conserve energy for bodily functions. This also happens when you overdo exercise as well. Generally, for most healthy women, you don't want to go lower than 1000 calories per day. For men, generally, you don't want to go lower than 1200 calories per day. The underlying problem with people that are dealing with this issue is a lack of trust in the process. So many of us have been indoctrinated to believe that fat is bad and eating the allotted macros and calories couldn't possibly result in weight loss. We have to trust the process and know that our success is coming through that process and not excessive exercise or a deep caloric deficit.

I don't want to beat a dead horse but, these issues can pretty much all be prevented through the tracking and measuring of the foods that you are eating. Again, I know that there are plenty of people that do not want to count and track, but I promise that it does help.

**The ninth piece of sisterly advice is to incorporate inter-mittent fasting into your weight loss plan _AFTER_ you have become fat adapted.**

Once your body gets used to burning fat for energy in-stead of glucose (carbs), it is said that you have become fat adapted. Your cravings for sugar and carbs have subsided, you've gotten past the keto flu and now you've got more en-ergy than you've had in a very long time. Where before, you had to stop and refuel with snacks heavy in carbs and sugar, you're able to go longer between meals without feeling hun-gry. When I reached this stage, my hunger, which used to scream at me "EAT...NOW", became just a nice little whis-per that would say "you know, we could eat...I mean, if you're not too busy....no rush...". It generally takes any-where from three to six weeks to get to this phase. This is the point in your journey to think about starting intermittent fasting to put your weight loss on warp speed.

Intermittent fasting is a meal timing system where you alternate between times of eating and times of fasting (not eating). In simple terms, it is the skipping of meal(s) (fasting period) until your desired eating window opens and then at that point, you'd eat (eating period).

The most common fasting cycle on intermittent fasting is 16/8. This means that an individual would fast for 16 hours of the day and their eating window would be open for 8 hours of the day. A practical illustration of this would be if you finished eating dinner tonight at 8 pm, you would then wait 16 hours until your next meal. You would then eat your next meal at 12 noon tomorrow. Because you have chosen an 8-hour eating window, you would finish eating your last meal at 8 pm tomorrow night. Most people like the 16/8 timing because they are asleep through most of the fast, so it's easy to start and stick with. You can adapt the timing as you need to. There are some people who practice 20/4 and even eat only one meal a day by practicing something like a 23/1.

During your fasting period you can drink unsweetened coffee, tea, water and no-calorie drinks to help take the edge off any hunger you may experience. I would not recommend taking in anything that has over 50 calories as it can cause an insulin response in the body, which defeats the point of the intermittent fasting process. There are easily accessible videos on YouTube that show that drinking bulletproof coffee will not break your fast, but I, personally, like to keep it on the safe side so I stick with water and black coffee during my fasting period.

The reason that intermittent fasting is an effective tool is that as we eat, our body produces insulin. As we reduce the number of times we eat daily, we are increasing our body's sensitivity to insulin. Then when we do eat, our bodies are much more likely to efficiently use the food that we eat for energy and muscle production, which promotes fat loss. Furthermore, human growth hormone is also released during fasting periods which can be very helpful for people who are concerned with muscle loss due to fasting. This infusion of human growth hormone primes muscles. With that, the reduction of insulin production basically turns the body into a fat furnace, especially during periods of fasted workouts.

One mistake that I made in my journey was to start the process of intermittent fasting too early in the process. I started before I was fat adapted; in fact, I have been doing intermittent fasting since day one. It was incredibly difficult and forced me to stretch my will at a level that was unnecessary, looking back on it. I made things harder than they needed to be. If I had one piece of advice for intermittent fasting, it would be to make life easier on yourself by waiting until you are fat adapted to start intermittent fasting. You will not have to fight your grumbling stomach, and potentially give in to the cravings and hunger.

I still practice intermittent fasting to this day. I do plan ahead on special occasions to move my eating window if there is an event that includes food or eating so that I can enjoy the time with my family and friends without compromising the goals I have set for myself.

**The tenth piece of sisterly advice is plan ahead if you can BUT, if an impromptu event pops up, enjoy the time with your friends and family. Get right back on your eating plan afterward.**

Look, I know exactly how hard it is to let go of your plan when a last-minute event or occasion pops up, but for many of us, the reason we embarked on this Keto journey was so that we could live a whole and healthy life. A part of living that whole and healthy life is enjoying the time we have with our family and friends so ENJOY IT! Try to make food choices that align as closely to your goals as possible but don't decline to spend that time with the important people in your life because of something as small as food or meal timing. If you make a choice that doesn't align with your goals, pick yourself up, dust yourself off, and start again on the next meal. I'll say it again, shake it off, drink some water, and move on. Don't go into an extreme fast or extreme exercise. You may end up doing more harm than good. Your success is on its way, just continue to work forward towards your goal.

# Chapter 8: Supplements

The final piece of sisterly advice is to keep your Keto as natural as possible.

I believe that you do not need to waste your money on teas, wraps, pills, potions, or lotions to get healthy and lose weight. In this section of the book, I will address frequently asked questions, but one of the most asked questions I get, which I feel deserves its own section, is the question about supplements that can be taken to either speed up the ketosis process or weight loss overall. Personally, I don't believe that getting some of these types of supplements are necessary to be successful on the Keto diet. I am not talking about vitamin or mineral supplements which I do encourage if you have a deficiency that you are unable to meet through eating whole foods. If I had to choose how to spend my dollars effectively, I would choose the best quality grass-fed/pasture fed meats, seafood, quality vegetables, avocado oil, good tasting olive oil, or a good keto cook book. The list below contains some of the popular keto supplements out there:

**Exogenous Ketones:** These are (basically) synthetic ketones that are produced outside of the body that you introduce in. Studies have been carried out, and it shows that these products are of similar molecular makeup of the ketones that the body produces. So, it can help to put you into a state of ketosis. They also offer appetite control and can help with keto flu as well.

**MCT Oil:** Medium Chain Triglyceride is a unique fat that cannot be stored by the body. They are either used for energy or released from the body. When it is taken, it goes directly to the liver from the small intestine and used for energy. Other benefits of MCT oil is that it can help with ketone production and appetite control and offers a natural energy boost.

**Collagen Peptides:** Collagen makes up around 30% of the protein in the body, and many of us associate this particular protein with the upkeep of our skin, hair and nails. The benefits of collagen peptides include stronger muscles and bones, more youthful skin, it can be used to help with inflammation issues, and can also help with appetite control as well.

**Magnesium:** If you are having a hard time getting magnesium through the eating of leafy green veggies like spinach and kale you can use a magnesium supplement to assist. A deficiency in magnesium can result in muscle cramps, spasms and fatigue.

**Fiber:** Because keto is a low carb lifestyle this can sometimes leave us deficient in fiber which is important to having healthy bowel movements and avoiding bloating and constipation. Chia seeds, flax seeds, and psyllium husks are all great sources of fiber.

**Fish Oil:** Omega 3 fatty acids are an essential fatty acid used to help make cell membranes and help to protect the brain, so it is very important to make sure that we get enough. Since we can't produce them on our own, it's important to get it through our diet from sources like fatty fish (salmon), avocados, chia seeds, and flax seeds or a good fish oil supplement.

As I get ready to close, I wanted to include some general frequently asked Keto questions.

*How is Keto different from Atkins?* Atkins and keto both start with the reduction of carbs down to 5% of the daily caloric intake but as time goes on, people on the Atkins plan will increase their carb intake to figure out the max that they can eat before they are kicked out of ketosis, while my fellow Keto-ers will remain at 5%. Atkins morphs into a low carb diet while keto is and remains a high healthy fat way of eating.

*How Long Does it take to get into ketosis?* It generally takes anywhere from 2 to 7 days to get into ketosis assuming you've reduced your carbs down to an appropriate level.

*Are ketoacidosis and ketosis the same?* No! ketoacidosis, is a life-threatening complication of type 1 diabetes. It comes as a result of extremely high levels of ketones and blood sugar. This condition attacks your vital organs (liver and kidneys) and requires immediate medical intervention. Meanwhile, ketosis is simply the presence of ketones, and these ketones are produced when the body burns stored fat.

*What will Keto do to my cholesterol levels?* If you are enjoying the keto lifestyle and losing weight, generally, your overall blood lipid levels should also begin to drop as well. However, your cholesterol levels will be dependent on the kinds of foods and types of fat you're eating. If you are sticking with good healthy fats found in avocados, avocado oil and olive oil, for example, instead of over doing it on butter and bacon, generally speaking, your cholesterol should be fine.

*If I eat too much protein will it be converted into glucose and therefore kick me out of ketosis?* No, and I wish that myth would die! Look, you need to meet your protein macro as protein is the substance through which bone, blood and body tissues are formed. There was a myth that has circulated, which says eating too much protein will result in gluconeogenesis, and that, in laymen's terms, is the body turning that protein into glucose and using that for energy instead of fat. Again, it is NOT TRUE. Meet your protein macro, and your body will thank you!

*Which Macro Should we meet – Fat, Protein, or Carbs?* You need to meet your protein macro, it is your goal macro. Your carb macro is a limit – not to be exceeded. In fact, the farther you stay away from it, the better. Your fat macro is the lever. It is the thing (along with your protein) that will keep you full and satisfied so that you will not want to snack between meals.

*How much weight can I lose with keto OR Can I lose ___ pounds by _____ date?* That is something that is dependent on so many factors that I couldn't even begin to name them in this book. Everyone's body is different, so I would call BS on anyone who can tell you how much weight you will lose in any amount of time. Do I believe that you can meet your weight loss goals, given enough time? Absolutely. Unfortunately, I, nor anyone else, can tell you accurately or definitively how much you will lose over a given period. Sorry!

***Is Keto a sustainable way of eating?*** Yes! What isn't sustainable about eating healthy whole foods – meats, vegetables, and healthy fats with an occasional treat with friends and family for special occasions and holidays? I'm convinced that the people that question its sustainability are the ones that have been misinformed by people who believe that Keto is all bacon, butter, MCT oil and processed meats, which it is not.

***What's the difference between 'strict Keto', 'Lazy Keto', and 'Dirty Keto'?*** Strict Keto follows the tenets explained in this book; carbs are kept at less than 20 net grams, you're avoiding highly processed foods choosing instead to eat whole foods, getting your carbs from mostly green leafy veggies, eliminating added sugar, counting and tracking food intake and macros. **Lazy Keto** is pretty much the same as above without the counting or tracking of your macros with the exception of carbs (for some people, others do not count or track anything). **Dirty Keto** is when you're eating anything that will fit your macros. So that means that the emphasis is not necessarily placed on eating whole foods, and there is no distinction between highly processed meats and fats and healthier options if there is room for it in your macros. By the way, I really dislike the negative connotation behind using the terms "dirty" and "lazy". If these are the ways that you are comfortable adjusting your eating habits to meet your weight loss and health goals, I say more power to you! You are neither lazy nor dirty!

***Can you drink alcohol on Keto?*** Yes, depending on the type of alcohol but keep in mind that overdoing it could hinder weight loss. Also, beware that after enjoying the Keto lifestyle for a while, your alcohol tolerance may be lower than it previously was, and your hangover could be worse. Stick with lower carb options such as Champagne, Red and white wine options. Liquor options include vodka, whisky, brandy, tequila and other pure alcohols.

## Closing Words

As I close this book, I want to take a second to thank you for reading. I want to open and honestly share not only my experience but, a bit of the research that I have done in an effort to make your experience of stepping into the keto lifestyle as easy and as seamless as possible. One thing that I have found is that it's not always easy to ask questions of people that have been there. In this age where information is power, there are some folks out there that will hoard information and only share it if you pay a fool's ransom for it. I have been openly sharing, not only the information in this book but also new information that I have found through researching the answers for questions asked on the My Sister's Keto podcast and via our social media pages. I believe that we all deserve to have access to the information that could have an impact on our health and, to that end, if there is ever any question that I can answer for you, please feel free to contact me via our website www.mysistersketo.com. You can also interact with me on social media. On Instagram, you can find me at @mysistersketodiet and there is also the Facebook group, My Sister's Keto, as well.

At the end of the day, I want us all to win! We all deserve good health and happiness. I pray that we all find the success that we seek. I know that if we change the way that we think about ourselves and how we think about the things we can accomplish, we can and will change our lives!

Good luck to you!

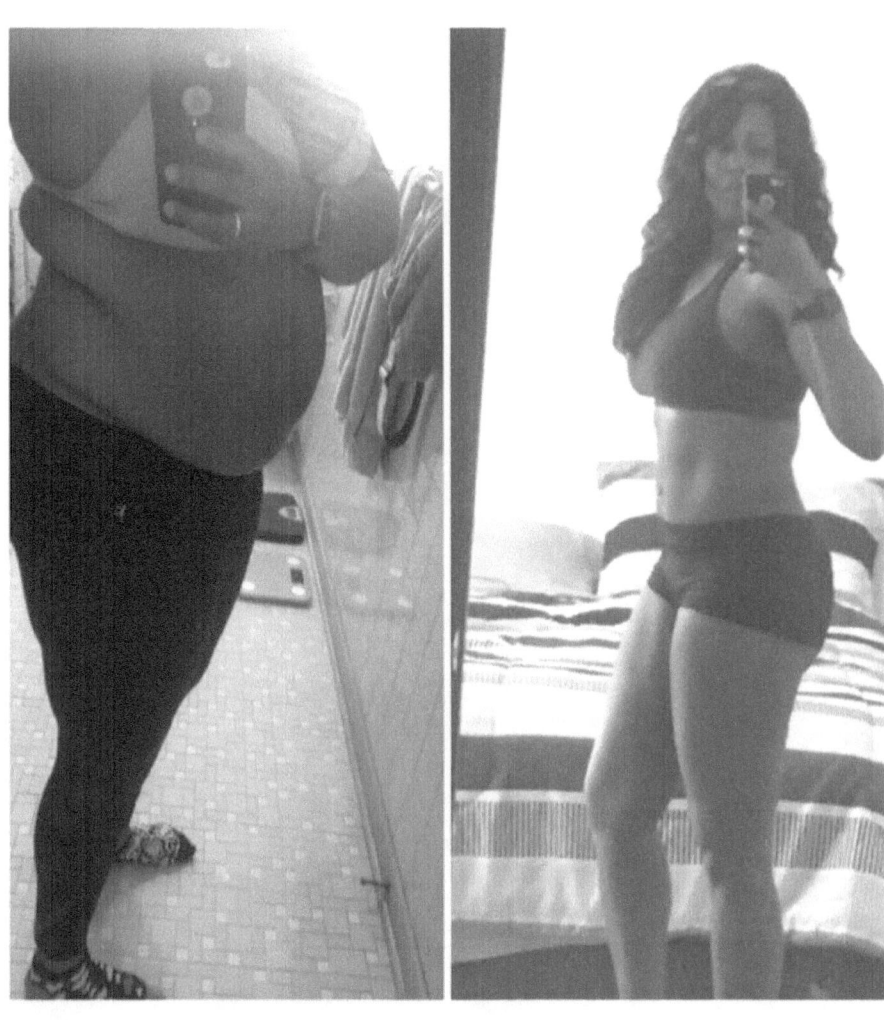